A – Z

Of

Crohn's Disease

Written by

Andrew D Beattie
www.AndrewDBeattie.co.uk[1]

---

1. http://www.AndrewDBeattie.co.uk

Table of Contents

Dedicated to:

This book is dedicated to all those who have faced the challenges of Crohn's Disease with courage, resilience, and unwavering determination.

To the individuals and their families who have navigated the unpredictable journey of this condition, you are the true heroes of this story.

May this book serve as a source of knowledge, support, and hope, as we strive for a world where Crohn's Disease is better understood and where those affected can live their lives to the fullest.

With heartfelt gratitude for your strength and inspiration,

Andrew D Beattie

Introduction

Welcome to "All About Crohn's Disease". As someone is personally affected by Crohn's disease, I understand the physical, emotional, and mental challenges that come with this condition. This book is a reflection of my journey and a comprehensive guide to understanding the many facets of this complex disease.

Crohn's disease, a type of inflammatory bowel disease, is a lifelong journey marked by periods of remission and flare-ups. It can affect any part of the gastrointestinal tract, making each person's experience unique.

In this book, we delve into the various types of Crohn's disease, its symptoms, diagnostic procedures, treatment options, and the latest research in the field. We also explore the often-overlooked aspect of mental health in dealing with Crohn's disease. Living with a chronic illness can take a toll on one's mental well-being, and it's crucial to address this aspect alongside physical health.

Whether you're newly diagnosed, a long-term fighter, a healthcare professional, or a loved one trying to provide support, "All About Crohn's Disease" aims to be your reliable companion. My goal is to empower you with knowledge and understanding, fostering resilience in the face of this challenging disease.

Join me as we navigate the world of Crohn's disease together. Let's transform complex medical jargon into accessible information and provide practical advice to manage and thrive despite the condition. Welcome aboard! Let's embark on this enlightening journey together.

Chapter 1: What is Crohn's Disease?

Crohn's disease is a chronic condition that causes inflammation and irritation in your digestive tract[1][2]. It is a type of inflammatory bowel disease (IBD) and can affect any part of the gastrointestinal tract, from your mouth to your anus[3][4][5]. However, it most commonly affects the small intestine and the beginning of the large intestine[6][7].

The inflammation caused by Crohn's disease often spreads into the deeper layers of the bowel, which can lead to life-threatening complications[8][9]. The symptoms of Crohn's disease can range from mild to severe and may develop gradually or come on suddenly, without warning[10][11]. You may also have periods of time when you have no signs or symptoms (remission) and periods when symptoms flare up[12][13].

---

1. https://www.niddk.nih.gov/health-information/digestive-diseases/crohns-disease/definition-facts

2. https://www.niddk.nih.gov/health-information/digestive-diseases/crohns-disease/definition-facts

3. https://www.mayoclinic.org/diseases-conditions/crohns-disease/symptoms-causes/syc-20353304

4. https://www.mayoclinic.org/diseases-conditions/crohns-disease/symptoms-causes/syc-20353304

5. https://www.niddk.nih.gov/health-information/digestive-diseases/crohns-disease/definition-facts

6. https://www.niddk.nih.gov/health-information/digestive-diseases/crohns-disease/definition-facts

7. https://www.niddk.nih.gov/health-information/digestive-diseases/crohns-disease/definition-facts

8. https://www.mayoclinic.org/diseases-conditions/crohns-disease/symptoms-causes/syc-20353304

9. https://www.mayoclinic.org/diseases-conditions/crohns-disease/symptoms-causes/syc-20353304

10. https://www.mayoclinic.org/diseases-conditions/crohns-disease/symptoms-causes/syc-20353304

11. https://www.mayoclinic.org/diseases-conditions/crohns-disease/symptoms-causes/syc-20353304

12. https://www.mayoclinic.org/diseases-conditions/crohns-disease/symptoms-causes/syc-20353304

The main symptoms of Crohn's disease include:

- **Diarrhea**: This happens when the intestines cannot absorb all the nutrients or fluid produced during the digestive process, causing stools to be loose and watery[14][15].

- **Abdominal pain and cramping**: This often occurs in the lower right area of your abdomen but can happen anywhere along the digestive tract. It can range from mild to severe, and may be constant or may come and go[16][17].

- **Blood in stool**: Chronic, constant inflammation from Crohn's disease can lead to ulcers, fistulas, and fissures throughout the digestive tract. These can cause bleeding to occur, particularly in the lower intestines and rectum[18][19].

- **Fatigue**: This is a common symptom and can be caused by the disease itself, by anemia due to blood loss, or by the side effects of medications[20][21].

- **Weight loss**: This can occur as a result of reduced appetite or malabsorption of nutrients due to inflammation in the intestines[22][23].

13.　　https://www.mayoclinic.org/diseases-conditions/crohns-disease/symptoms-causes/syc-20353304

14. https://www.msn.com/en-us/health/condition/Crohn

15. https://www.msn.com/en-us/health/condition/Crohn

16. https://www.msn.com/en-us/health/condition/Crohn

17. https://www.msn.com/en-us/health/condition/Crohn

18. https://www.msn.com/en-us/health/condition/Crohn

19. https://www.msn.com/en-us/health/condition/Crohn

20. https://www.msn.com/en-us/health/condition/Crohn

21. https://www.msn.com/en-us/health/condition/Crohn

22. https://www.msn.com/en-us/health/condition/Crohn

23. https://www.msn.com/en-us/health/condition/Crohn

The exact cause of Crohn's disease is unknown. It's thought several things could play a role, including your genes (you're more likely to get it if a close family member has it), a problem with the immune system that causes it to attack the digestive system, smoking, a previous stomach bug, an abnormal balance of gut bacteria[24][25].

Diagnosis involves physical examination, lab tests and imaging tests to ascertain the condition and severity of the disease. These tests may include physical examination to check for possible causes of the symptoms, complete blood count (CBC), CT scan of the abdomen, endoscopy, barium swallow[26][27].

There is no known cure for Crohn's disease, but therapies can greatly reduce its signs and symptoms and even bring about long-term remission and healing of inflammation. With treatment, many people with Crohn's disease are able to function well[28][29].

Learn more:
1. niddk.nih.gov[30] 2. mayoclinic.org[31] 3. msn.com[32] 4. nhs.uk[33] 5. msn.com[34]

---

24.   https://www.nhs.uk/conditions/crohns-disease/

25.   https://www.nhs.uk/conditions/crohns-disease/

26.   https://www.msn.com/en-us/health/condition/Crohn

27.   https://www.msn.com/en-us/health/condition/Crohn

28.   https://www.mayoclinic.org/diseases-conditions/crohns-disease/symptoms-causes/
     syc-20353304

29.   https://www.mayoclinic.org/diseases-conditions/crohns-disease/symptoms-causes/
     syc-20353304

30.   https://www.niddk.nih.gov/health-information/digestive-diseases/crohns-disease/definition-facts

31.   https://www.mayoclinic.org/diseases-conditions/crohns-disease/symptoms-causes/syc-20353304

32.   https://www.msn.com/en-us/health/condition/Crohn

33.   https://www.nhs.uk/conditions/crohns-disease/

34.   https://www.msn.com/en-us/health/condition/Crohn's-disease/hp-Crohn's-disease?source=conditioncdx

Types of Crohn's Disease There are five types of Crohn's disease, each affecting different parts of the digestive tract:

1. **Ileocolitis and ileitis**: Inflammation and irritation of the ileum (the lower part of the small intestine) and colon.
2. **Gastroduodenal Crohn's disease**: Affects the stomach and duodenum (the first part of the small intestine).
3. **Jejunoileitis**: Occurs in the jejunum, or the second part of the small intestine.
4. **Granulomatous colitis**: Affects only the colon (the main part of the large intestine).

Main Symptoms The main symptoms of Crohn's disease are diarrhoea, stomach aches and cramps, blood in your stool, tiredness (fatigue), and weight loss.

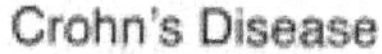

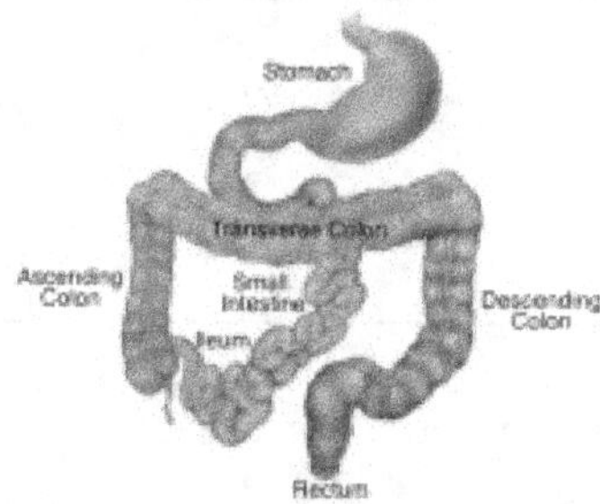

Chapter 2: Prevalence and Demographics

Crohn's Disease can affect individuals of any age, but it most commonly begins in young adults between the ages of 15 and 35. While the exact cause of Crohn's Disease is not fully understood, it is believed to result from a combination of genetic, environmental, and immune system factors. Here's a breakdown of who may be more prone to developing Crohn's Disease and some of the potential contributing factors:

1. Genetic Predisposition: There is a significant genetic component to Crohn's Disease. Individuals with a family history of the condition are at a higher risk. Specific genes, such as NOD2, have been associated with an increased susceptibility to Crohn's.

2. Immune System: It is thought that Crohn's Disease may result from an abnormal immune response to certain microorganisms or bacteria in the digestive tract. The immune system, in trying to fight off perceived threats, causes inflammation in the GI tract.

3. Environmental Factors: While genetics play a role, environmental factors are also believed to contribute. Factors such as diet, smoking, and exposure to certain infections or antibiotics may influence the risk of developing Crohn's Disease. For example, smoking is associated with a higher risk of developing Crohn's.

4. Autoimmune Component: Crohn's Disease is considered an autoimmune disorder, where the immune system mistakenly attacks healthy cells in the digestive tract. Autoimmune diseases often have a genetic predisposition and are triggered by environmental factors.

5. Geography: There are geographical differences in the prevalence of Crohn's Disease, with higher rates reported in Western countries. This suggests that environmental factors, including diet and lifestyle, may play a role.

It's important to note that while these factors may increase the risk of developing Crohn's Disease, they do not guarantee its onset. Likewise, someone without known risk factors can still develop the condition.

Crohn's Disease is a complex and multifactorial condition, and researchers are continually studying its causes and triggers.

If you suspect you may have Crohn's Disease or are concerned about your risk due to a family history or other factors, it's essential to consult with a healthcare professional for a proper evaluation, diagnosis, and personalized guidance on managing the condition. Early detection and appropriate management can help improve the quality of life for individuals with Crohn's Disease.

United Kingdom:

- Gender: The disease appears to affect men and women roughly equally[1][2].
- Age: The prevalence of Crohn's or Colitis increases to 1 in every 67 for people aged over 70[3][4].
- Race: The prevalence of Crohn's and Colitis was higher in people who declared their ethnicity as white compared with all other ethnicity groups[5][6].

USA:

- Gender: In the United States, ulcerative colitis is slightly more common in males, while Crohn's disease is more frequent in females[7][8].

1. https://www.verywellhealth.com/crohns-disease-age-of-onset-5214471

2. https://www.verywellhealth.com/crohns-disease-age-of-onset-5214471

3. https://journals.plos.org/plosone/article?id=10.1371/journal.pone.0252458

4. https://journals.plos.org/plosone/article?id=10.1371/journal.pone.0252458

5. https://journals.plos.org/plosone/article?id=10.1371/journal.pone.0252458

6. https://journals.plos.org/plosone/article?id=10.1371/journal.pone.0252458

7. https://academic.oup.com/ibdjournal/article/12/10/936/4682843

8. https://academic.oup.com/ibdjournal/article/12/10/936/4682843

- Age: A higher percentage of adults aged 45–64 (1.5%) and ≥65 (1.7%) years had IBD compared with adults aged 18–24 (0.5%) and 25–44 (1.0%) years[9][10].
- Race: IBD was found in 1.4 percent of non-Hispanic white people, 0.6 percent of non-Hispanic Black people, 1.2 percent of Hispanics, and 0.8 percent among all other non-Hispanic adults[11][12].

Canada:

- Gender: The disease appears to affect men and women roughly equally[13][14].
- Age: Inflammatory bowel disease affects all age groups with adolescents and young adults at highest risk of diagnosis.
- Race: Canadians of all ethnicities are being diagnosed with IBD including known high-risk groups such as Ashkenazi Jews and offspring of South Asian immigrants who were previously thought to be low risk.

Australia:

---

9. https://publichealth.massey.ac.nz/home/research/research-projects/the-epidemiology-of-crohn-s-and-colitis-in-new-zealand-a-data-linkage-study/

10. https://publichealth.massey.ac.nz/home/research/research-projects/the-epidemiology-of-crohn-s-and-colitis-in-new-zealand-a-data-linkage-study/

11. https://www.moh.govt.nz/notebook/nbbooks.nsf/0/41CA23E0176F0B8DCC257A4E007C1F71/$file/surveillance-increased-risk-colorectal-cancer.pdf

12. https://www.moh.govt.nz/notebook/nbbooks.nsf/0/41CA23E0176F0B8DCC257A4E007C1F71/$file/surveillance-increased-risk-colorectal-cancer.pdf

13. https://www.verywellhealth.com/crohns-disease-age-of-onset-5214471

14. https://www.verywellhealth.com/crohns-disease-age-of-onset-5214471

- Gender: The disease appears to affect men and women roughly equally[15][16]. Males were independently associated with a lower risk of Crohn's disease but a greater risk of ulcerative colitis than females[17][18].

- Age: The age standardised IBD prevalence rate was found to be 348 cases per 100,000 population. Its prevalence was higher in older people: 612 per 100,000 people aged 65 years or more and 891 per 100,000 people aged 85 years or more[19][20]. About 25% of people with Crohn's disease will develop it as children or young adults before the age of 20. Most cases, however, occur between the ages of 20 and 30[21][22]. Crohn's can occur at any age, but most people are diagnosed between the ages of 15 and 30[23][24].

- Race: Other factors positively associated with both Crohn's disease and ulcerative colitis were age (≥ 25 years), non-Indigenous status and socioeconomic advantage[25][26].

15. https://www.verywellhealth.com/crohns-disease-age-of-onset-5214471

16. https://www.verywellhealth.com/crohns-disease-age-of-onset-5214471

17. https://www.verywellhealth.com/crohns-disease-age-of-onset-5214471

18. https://journals.plos.org/plosone/article?id=10.1371/journal.pone.0252458

19. https://www.mja.com.au/journal/2021/214/8/high-prevalence-crohn-disease-and-ulcerative-colitis-among-older-people-sydney

20. https://www.mja.com.au/journal/2021/214/8/high-prevalence-crohn-disease-and-ulcerative-colitis-among-older-people-sydney

21. https://www.verywellhealth.com/crohns-disease-age-of-onset-5214471

22. https://www.verywellhealth.com/crohns-disease-age-of-onset-5214471

23. https://www.verywellhealth.com/crohns-disease-age-of-onset-5214471

24. https://www.hudson.org.au/news/crohns-disease-in-australia-the-latest-research/

25. https://journals.plos.org/plosone/article?id=10.1371/journal.pone.0252458

26. https://journals.plos.org/plosone/article?id=10.1371/journal.pone.0252458

New Zealand:

- Gender: Both Crohn's disease and ulcerative colitis have a peak incidence in people aged between 18 and 35 years, with a second peak of ulcerative colitis between age 60–70 years, although IBD can present in people of any age[27,28]. CD patients were more likely than UC patients to be female (61.4% vs. 47.1%) and to be younger (median age, 39.9 years vs. 43.7 years)[29,30].
- Age: IBD affects people of all ages but is primarily a disease of young adults in the prime of their lives, with onset typically between the ages of 15-35[31,32].
- Race: In an analysis of IBD in the Otago region, only 1.8% of cases were in people of Māori ethnicity, despite this group accounting for 7.5% of the Otago population[33,10,34].

Please note that these statistics might have changed as my information was updated in 2021, and the prevalence of Crohn's disease can vary over time due to many factors such as changes in lifestyle, diet, and healthcare practices.

Learn more:

---

27. https://bpac.org.nz/2021/ibd.aspx

28. https://bpac.org.nz/2021/ibd.aspx

29. https://www.verywellhealth.com/crohns-disease-age-of-onset-5214471

30. https://academic.oup.com/ibdjournal/article/12/10/936/4682843

31. https://www.verywellhealth.com/crohns-disease-age-of-onset-5214471

32. https://www.healthpoint.co.nz/community-health-and-social-services/community-health/crohns-and-colitis-new-zealand-1/

33. https://bpac.org.nz/2021/docs/ibd.pdf

34. https://bpac.org.nz/2021/docs/ibd.pdf

1. verywellhealth.com[35] 2. journals.plos.org[36] 3. academic.oup.com[37] 4. publichealth.massey.ac.nz[38] 5. moh.govt.nz[39] 6. mja.com.au[40] 7. hudson.org.au[41] 8. bpac.org.nz[42] 9. healthpoint.co.nz[43] 10. bpac.org.nz[44] 11.mycrohnsandcolitisteam.com[45] 12. verywellhealth.com[46] 13.hrc.govt.nz[47] 14. symbiosisonlinepublishing.com[48] 15. doi.org[49] 16. moh.govt.nz[50]

35.	https://www.verywellhealth.com/crohns-disease-age-of-onset-5214471

36.	https://journals.plos.org/plosone/article?id=10.1371/journal.pone.0252458

37.	https://academic.oup.com/ibdjournal/article/12/10/936/4682843

38.	https://publichealth.massey.ac.nz/home/research/research-projects/the-epidemiology-of-crohn-s-and-colitis-in-new-zealand-a-data-linkage-study/

39.	https://www.moh.govt.nz/notebook/nbbooks.nsf/0/41CA23E0176F0B8DCC257A4E007C1F71/$file/surveillance-increased-risk-colorectal-cancer.pdf

40.	https://www.mja.com.au/journal/2021/214/8/high-prevalence-crohn-disease-and-ulcerative-colitis-among-older-people-sydney

41.	https://www.hudson.org.au/news/crohns-disease-in-australia-the-latest-research/

42.	https://bpac.org.nz/2021/ibd.aspx

43.	https://www.healthpoint.co.nz/community-health-and-social-services/community-health/crohns-and-colitis-new-zealand-1/

44.	https://bpac.org.nz/2021/docs/ibd.pdf

45.	https://www.mycrohnsandcolitisteam.com/resources/who-gets-crohns-and-colitis-ibd-across-racial-and-ethnic-groups

46.	https://www.verywellhealth.com/crohn-s-disease-facts-5324626

47.	https://www.hrc.govt.nz/resources/research-repository/epidemiology-crohns-and-colitis-new-zealand-data-linkage-study

48.	https://symbiosisonlinepublishing.com/immunology/immunology25.php

49.	https://doi.org/10.1371/journal.pone.0252458

50.	https://www.moh.govt.nz/notebook/nbbooks.nsf/0/41CA23E0176F0B8DCC257A4E007C1F71/

Chapter 3: Historical Perspective and Discovery

In order to understand the current state of knowledge about Crohn's Disease, it's important to delve into its historical context and the journey of its discovery.

Ancient Observations: Crohn's Disease is not a recent discovery but rather a condition that has affected humans for centuries. In ancient writings from as far back as the 3rd century BC, there are descriptions of individuals experiencing symptoms consistent with what we now recognize as Crohn's Disease. These writings mention chronic abdominal pain, diarrhoea, and digestive discomfort.

Early Medical Accounts: During the 19th and early 20th centuries, physicians and surgeons began to document cases that closely resembled what we now call Crohn's Disease. However, it was often confused with other gastrointestinal disorders due to limited medical understanding at the time.

Breakthrough in the 20th Century: The critical turning point in understanding Crohn's Disease occurred in the early 20th century when three physicians independently made significant contributions to its recognition and description.

1. Burrill Bernard Crohn: In 1932, Dr. Burrill Bernard Crohn, along with Dr. Leon Ginzburg and Dr. Gordon D. Oppenheimer, published a seminal paper in the Journal of the American Medical Association. This paper outlined the distinct characteristics of a new disease they called "Terminal Ileitis." They described the inflammation and ulceration of the small intestine, which we now know as a hallmark of Crohn's Disease. Consequently, the condition was named after Dr. Crohn in recognition of his pioneering work.

2. Historical Significance of the Description:

◈ Dr. Crohn's work was groundbreaking because it separated this condition from other digestive disorders, providing a clearer understanding of its distinct features.

◈ The recognition of Crohn's Disease led to further research and the development of diagnostic criteria.

Advancements in Diagnosis and Treatment:

◈ The identification of Crohn's Disease paved the way for improved diagnostic techniques, such as endoscopy and imaging, which allow doctors to visualize the inflamed areas of the gastrointestinal tract.

◈ Over the years, medical research has led to the development of medications and surgical interventions to manage the disease and improve the quality of life for those affected.

Recognition of Its Complexity: Crohn's Disease has since been recognized as a complex condition with a wide range of symptoms and potential complications. It is not merely a gastrointestinal disorder but also has immunological and genetic components.

Conclusion: Understanding the historical perspective of Crohn's Disease highlights the progress that has been made in recognizing and addressing this condition. The pioneering work of Dr. Burrill Bernard Crohn and his colleagues laid the foundation for ongoing research, improved treatments, and better support for individuals living with Crohn's Disease.

In the following chapters, we will delve deeper into the clinical aspects of Crohn's Disease, its causes, symptoms, and the various approaches to managing and living with this condition.

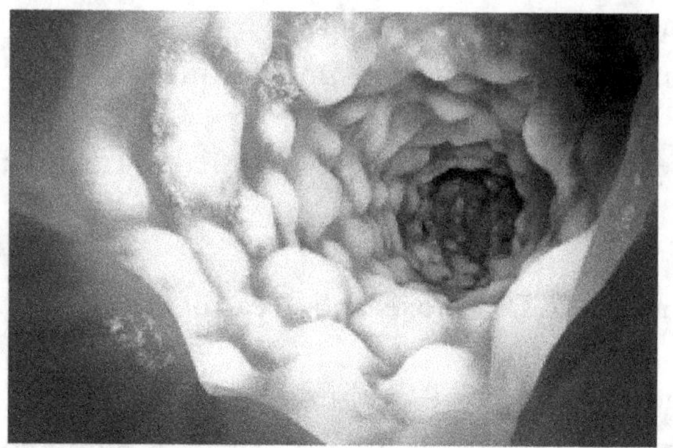

Chapter 4: Understanding the Digestive System

To comprehend the intricacies of Crohn's Disease, it's essential to first grasp the fundamental workings of the digestive system, including how digestion takes place and the critical role of the immune system within the gut.

Overview of the Gastrointestinal Tract: The gastrointestinal (GI) tract, often referred to as the digestive tract, is a marvel of biological engineering. It is a long, hollow tube that begins at the mouth and extends to the anus, with several key components:

1. Mouth:

⬥ The digestive process commences in the mouth with the intake of food.

⬥ Salivary glands produce saliva, which contains enzymes that begin breaking down carbohydrates.

2. Oesophagus:

⬥ After chewing and swallowing, food travels down the oesophagus, a muscular tube that connects the mouth to the stomach.

3. Stomach:

⬥ In the stomach, food is mixed with gastric juices, which contain hydrochloric acid and enzymes.

⬥ This acidic environment helps further break down food and initiate protein digestion.

4. Small Intestine:

◈ Most of the digestion and nutrient absorption occur in the small intestine.

◈ The pancreas releases digestive enzymes, and the liver produces bile to assist in the breakdown of fats.

◈ Villi and microvilli in the small intestine increase the surface area for nutrient absorption.

5. Large Intestine (Colon):

◈ The remaining, indigestible material passes into the large intestine, where water and electrolytes are absorbed.

◈ The colon also houses beneficial gut bacteria that aid in the fermentation of certain substances.

How Digestion Works: Digestion is a complex process involving mechanical and chemical actions:

1. Mechanical Digestion:

◈ Begins in the mouth with chewing, which breaks food into smaller pieces.

◈ Continues in the stomach through muscular contractions that mix food with gastric juices.

◈ In the small intestine, segmentation movements further break down food and mix it with digestive enzymes.

2. Chemical Digestion:

◈ Enzymes from various digestive organs, including the mouth, stomach, pancreas, and small intestine, break down complex nutrients (carbohydrates, proteins, and fats) into simpler forms for absorption.

Role of the Immune System in the Gut:

◈ The gut is home to a vast and complex immune system that plays a crucial role in maintaining a balance between defence against pathogens and tolerance to beneficial microorganisms and food.

◈ Specialized immune cells, such as lymphocytes and macrophages, are present in the gut lining and gut-associated lymphoid tissue (GALT).

◈ The gut immune system actively monitors and responds to threats, including pathogens and potentially harmful substances from the diet.

Conclusion: A basic understanding of the gastrointestinal tract, the processes of digestion, and the role of the immune system within the gut is essential for comprehending how Crohn's Disease impacts this intricate system. In subsequent chapters, we will explore how disruptions in these processes can lead to the development and progression of Crohn's Disease and how this knowledge informs its management and treatment.

Chapter 5: Symptoms and Diagnosis

Recognizing the symptoms of Crohn's Disease and obtaining an accurate diagnosis are crucial steps in effectively managing this condition.

Common Symptoms of Crohn's Disease: Crohn's Disease can manifest with a range of symptoms, which can vary in intensity and may come and go. Common symptoms include:

1. Abdominal Pain: Persistent or intermittent abdominal pain, often in the lower right abdomen, is a hallmark of Crohn's Disease. The pain can be crampy and severe.

2. Diarrhoea: Frequent diarrhoea is a common symptom, which may be watery or contain blood and mucus.

3. Fatigue: Chronic inflammation and malabsorption of nutrients can lead to fatigue and general weakness.

4. Weight Loss: Unintended weight loss is often observed due to reduced appetite, malabsorption, and increased energy expenditure from inflammation.

5. Reduced Appetite: Many individuals with Crohn's Disease experience a loss of appetite, leading to decreased food intake.

6. Perianal Symptoms: Some people may have perianal symptoms, including fistulas (abnormal connections between the intestines and other organs), abscesses (collections of pus), or anal fissures.

7. Bowel Urgency: A strong urge to have a bowel movement is common, often leading to frequent visits to the restroom.

8. Nausea and Vomiting: Nausea and occasional vomiting can occur, particularly during flares.

9. Joint Pain: Joint pain and inflammation, known as arthralgia or arthritis, can affect individuals with Crohn's Disease.

10. Skin Issues: Skin problems such as rashes, ulcers, and erythema nodosum (painful red nodules) may be associated with Crohn's Disease.

The Diagnostic Process: Obtaining an accurate diagnosis of Crohn's Disease typically involves several steps:

1. Medical History: Your healthcare provider will take a detailed medical history, including your symptoms, their duration, and any family history of gastrointestinal disorders.

2. Physical Examination: A physical exam may reveal signs such as abdominal tenderness, weight loss, or perianal abnormalities.

3. Blood Tests: Blood tests can help identify signs of inflammation, anaemia, and nutritional deficiencies.

4. Stool Tests: Stool samples may be examined for signs of infection or inflammation.

5. Imaging Studies:

◈ **Endoscopy:** Colonoscopy and upper endoscopy are common procedures. They involve inserting a flexible tube with a camera into the digestive tract to visualize the lining, take biopsies, and assess the extent of inflammation.

◈ **Imaging:** Radiological studies like CT scans and MRIs can provide detailed images of the digestive tract, helping to locate areas of inflammation, strictures, or fistulas.

Biopsies: During endoscopy, tissue samples (biopsies) are often taken for microscopic examination to confirm the diagnosis and rule out other conditions.

Conclusion: Recognizing the common symptoms of Crohn's Disease and undergoing a thorough diagnostic process is crucial for timely and accurate diagnosis. The combination of medical history, physical examination, blood tests, stool tests, imaging studies, and biopsies allows healthcare providers to make an informed diagnosis and develop an appropriate treatment plan. In the following chapters, we will delve into the various aspects of managing Crohn's Disease, including treatment options and strategies for improving quality of life.

Chapter 6: Types and Location of Crohn's Disease

Crohn's Disease is a complex condition that can affect different parts of the gastrointestinal tract, and its presentation can vary from person to person.

Different Patterns and Locations of Inflammation:

Crohn's Disease is known for its ability to involve various segments of the gastrointestinal (GI) tract, leading to different patterns and locations of inflammation. The following are some common patterns:

1. Ileocolitis:

⬦ This is the most common form of Crohn's Disease and primarily affects the junction of the ileum (the last part of the small intestine) and the colon.

⬦ Symptoms often include right lower abdominal pain, diarrhoea, and weight loss.

2. Ileitis:

⬦ In this pattern, inflammation is limited to the ileum, without affecting the colon.

⬦ Symptoms may include abdominal pain and diarrhoea.

3. Colitis:

⬦ Some individuals with Crohn's Disease have inflammation that is confined to the colon.

⬦ Symptoms resemble those of ulcerative colitis, including abdominal pain and bloody diarrhoea.

4. Gastroduodenal Crohn's Disease:

◇ In rare cases, Crohn's Disease can affect the stomach and the beginning of the small intestine (duodenum).

◇ Symptoms may include nausea, vomiting, and upper abdominal pain.

5. Jejunoileitis:

◇ This pattern involves inflammation of the upper part of the small intestine (jejunum) and the ileum.

◇ Symptoms can include abdominal cramps and nutrient malabsorption.

Complications and Their Impact:

Crohn's Disease can lead to various complications, and their impact on an individual's health and quality of life can be significant:

1. Fistulas:

◇ Fistulas are abnormal connections or tunnels that can form between different parts of the GI tract or between the GI tract and other organs.

◇ They can cause pain, abscesses, and can complicate treatment.

2. Strictures:

◇ Inflammation and scarring can lead to the narrowing of the GI tract, known as strictures.

◇ Strictures can cause bowel obstruction, leading to severe abdominal pain and vomiting.

3. Abscesses:

◇ Pockets of pus (abscesses) can develop within the abdominal cavity, causing intense pain, fever, and a risk of systemic infection.

4. Perianal Complications:

◇ Perianal issues such as fistulas, abscesses, and anal fissures can be both painful and challenging to manage.

5. Malnutrition:

◇ Chronic inflammation and impaired nutrient absorption can lead to malnutrition, weight loss, and nutritional deficiencies.

6. Increased Cancer Risk:

◇ Long-term inflammation may increase the risk of colorectal cancer in individuals with Crohn's Disease, particularly if the colon is involved.

7. Psychosocial Impact:

◇ The chronic nature of Crohn's Disease, along with its symptoms and complications, can have a profound psychosocial impact, leading to stress, anxiety, and depression.

Conclusion: Understanding the different patterns and locations of Crohn's Disease inflammation is crucial for tailoring treatment approaches. Additionally, recognizing and addressing complications promptly is vital to improving the quality of life for individuals living with this condition. In the following chapters, we will explore various treatment options and strategies to manage and mitigate the impact of Crohn's Disease and its complications.

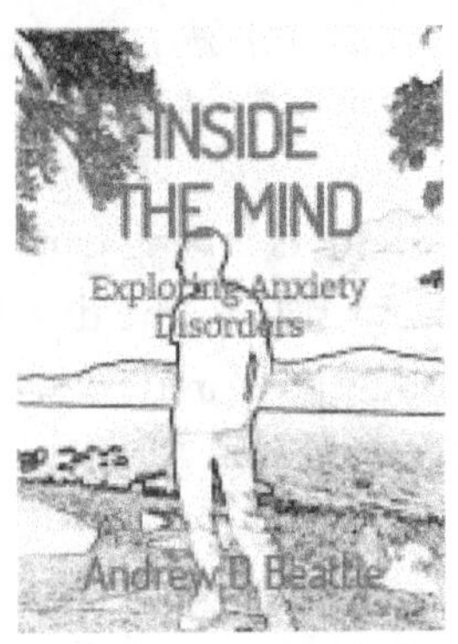

Chapter 7: Causes and Risk Factors

Crohn's Disease is a multifactorial condition influenced by a combination of genetic, environmental, and microbial factors. Understanding these causes and risk factors is essential for unravelling the complexities of the disease.

1. **Genetic Factors:** There is strong evidence to suggest that genetics play a significant role in the development of Crohn's Disease. Here are key points related to genetic factors:

2. **1. Family History:** Individuals with a family history of Crohn's Disease are at a higher risk of developing the condition. Having a first-degree relative (parent, sibling, or child) with Crohn's Disease increases the risk even further.

3. **2. Specific Genes:** Multiple genetic variants have been associated with Crohn's Disease, with the NOD2/CARD15 gene being one of the most extensively studied. Variations in this gene are more common in individuals with Crohn's Disease and can increase susceptibility.

4. **3. Complex Genetics:** Crohn's Disease is considered a complex genetic disorder, meaning that it involves multiple genes, each contributing a small part to the overall risk. Interactions between these genes and environmental factors are also believed to play a role.

5. **Environmental Influences:** While genetics set the stage, environmental factors are thought to trigger or exacerbate Crohn's Disease. Here are some environmental influences to consider:

6. **1. Diet:** Diet plays a crucial role in Crohn's Disease. Certain dietary factors, such as high consumption of processed foods, sugar, and unhealthy fats, have been associated with an increased risk. Conversely, diets rich in fruits, vegetables, and fibre may have a protective effect.

7. **2. Smoking:** Smoking is a well-established environmental risk factor for Crohn's Disease. It not only increases the risk of developing the disease but also worsens its course and reduces the effectiveness of treatment.

8. **3. Infections:** Some researchers believe that certain infections, particularly in childhood, may contribute to the development of Crohn's Disease. The gut microbiome's response to infections is a subject of ongoing research.

9. **The Role of the Microbiome:** The gut microbiome, the diverse community of microorganisms living in the digestive tract, is increasingly recognized as a key player in Crohn's Disease. Here's how it is involved:

10. **1. Dysbiosis:** Crohn's Disease is associated with an altered gut microbiome, characterized by a shift in the balance of beneficial and harmful bacteria.

11. **2. Immune Dysregulation:** Dysbiosis in the gut can trigger an abnormal immune response, leading to chronic inflammation characteristic of Crohn's Disease.

12. **3. Microbial Triggers:** Specific pathogens or alterations in the microbiome composition may serve as triggers for the development of the disease, especially in genetically predisposed individuals

Conclusion: Crohn's Disease is a complex condition influenced by genetic factors, environmental influences, and interactions with the gut microbiome. While genetic predisposition is an important factor, the interplay of these elements is what makes Crohn's Disease a multifaceted and challenging condition to understand and manage. In the subsequent chapters, we will explore strategies for managing and mitigating the impact of Crohn's Disease, considering the various factors involved in its development and progression.

Chapter 8: Treatment Options for Crohn's Disease

Managing Crohn's Disease involves a multifaceted approach that includes medications, biologics, immunosuppressants, and, in some cases, surgical interventions. This chapter explores the various treatment options available to individuals living with Crohn's Disease.

Medications for Crohn's Disease:

1. Aminosalicylates: These medications, such as mesalamine and sulfasalazine, are often used to treat mild to moderate cases of Crohn's Disease. They work by reducing inflammation in the gastrointestinal tract.

2. Corticosteroids: Prednisone and other corticosteroids can help control inflammation during flares. However, they are not suitable for long-term use due to potential side effects, including bone density loss, weight gain, and mood swings.

3. Immunomodulators: Medications like azathioprine and 6-mercaptopurine can help control the immune system's response, reducing inflammation in the gut. They are often used in combination with other treatments.

4. Biologics: Biologic drugs, such as infliximab, adalimumab, and vedolizumab, target specific proteins involved in the inflammatory process. They are used for moderate to severe cases and can induce and maintain remission.

5. Anti-diarrheal Agents: Medications like loperamide can help manage diarrhoea, a common symptom of Crohn's Disease.

6. Pain Relievers: Over-the-counter pain relievers like acetaminophen may help alleviate abdominal pain. However, non-steroidal anti-inflammatory drugs (NSAIDs) should be avoided due to their potential to worsen symptoms.

Biologics and Immunosuppressants:

1. Biologics: Biologic drugs are a significant advancement in Crohn's Disease treatment. They target specific molecules involved in inflammation. Common biologics include:

◇ **Anti-TNF Agents:** Examples include infliximab, adalimumab, and certolizumab pegol. They block tumour necrosis factor-alpha (TNF-alpha), a key inflammatory molecule.

◇ **Anti-IL-12/23 Agents:** Ustekinumab is an example, which targets interleukin-12 and -23.

◇ **Integrin Antagonists:** Vedolizumab is an integrin antagonist that works by selectively blocking gut-specific immune responses.

2. Immunosuppressants: These drugs suppress the immune system's activity to reduce inflammation. Common immunosuppressants include azathioprine, 6-mercaptopurine, and methotrexate. They are often used in combination with other treatments, especially in cases of steroid dependence or to maintain remission.

Surgical Interventions:

Surgery may be necessary in certain situations, especially when complications or severe symptoms arise:

1. Strictureplasty: This surgical procedure widens narrowed sections of the intestine (strictures) without removing any bowel.

2. Bowel Resection: In cases of severely damaged or obstructed intestine, a portion of the affected bowel may need to be removed. The healthy ends are then reconnected.

3. Fistula Repair: Surgery can be performed to close fistulas (abnormal connections between different parts of the intestine or between the intestine and other organs).

4. Temporary or Permanent Ostomy: In severe cases where intestinal function cannot be restored, a stoma may be created, allowing waste to exit the body into a bag. This can be temporary or permanent.

Combination Therapy: In many cases, a combination of treatments is used to manage Crohn's Disease effectively. This approach may involve using medications, biologics, and lifestyle modifications tailored to the individual's specific needs and disease severity.

Conclusion: The treatment of Crohn's Disease is highly individualized and depends on factors such as disease location, severity, and response to previous therapies. Close collaboration with healthcare providers is essential to develop a treatment plan that addresses symptoms, promotes remission, and improves the overall quality of life for individuals living with Crohn's Disease. Regular follow-up and adjustments to the treatment plan are often necessary to manage this chronic condition effectively.

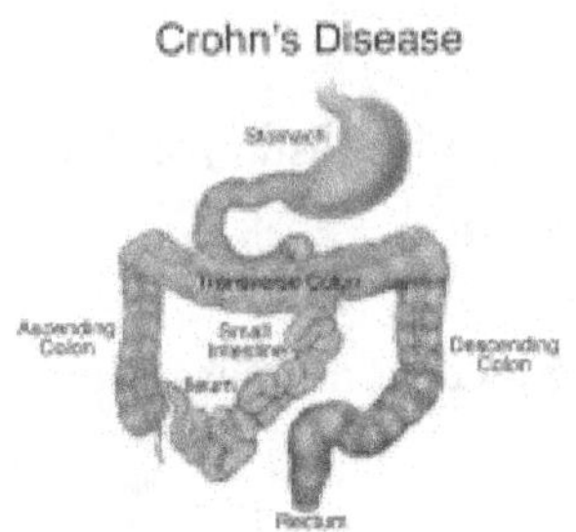

Chapter 9: Diet and Nutrition in Crohn's Disease

Diet plays a significant role in managing Crohn's Disease symptoms and promoting overall health. This chapter explores dietary triggers, considerations during flares and remission, and special diets tailored to the needs of individuals with Crohn's Disease.

Dietary Triggers and Considerations:

1. Trigger Foods: While the specific dietary triggers can vary from person to person, some common trigger foods and substances include:

◇ **High-Fiber Foods:** Rough or insoluble fibre found in certain fruits, vegetables, and whole grains can be challenging to digest and may aggravate symptoms during flares.

◇ **Dairy Products:** Lactose intolerance is common among individuals with Crohn's Disease, so dairy products may cause gas, bloating, and diarrhoea.

◇ **Fatty or Fried Foods:** High-fat foods can worsen diarrhoea and abdominal discomfort.

◇ **Spicy Foods:** Spices and seasonings may irritate the digestive tract.

◇ **Alcohol and Caffeine:** These can be dehydrating and may exacerbate diarrhoea.

2. Individual Sensitivities: It's crucial for individuals with Crohn's Disease to identify their specific trigger foods through a process of trial and error. Keeping a food journal can help pinpoint problematic items.

3. Nutrient Deficiencies: Chronic inflammation and malabsorption of nutrients can lead to deficiencies in vitamins and minerals, including vitamin B12, vitamin D, calcium, and iron. Regular monitoring and supplementation may be necessary.

Managing Nutrition During Flares and Remission:

1. During Flares:

◈ **Low-Residue Diet:** During flares, a low-residue diet that limits high-fibre foods can help reduce bowel movements and minimize irritation. It includes well-cooked, peeled, and seeded fruits and vegetables, tender meats, and refined grains.

◈ **Nutritional Supplements:** Liquid or semi-solid nutritional supplements can provide essential nutrients when it's challenging to eat regular meals.

2. During Remission:

◈ **Balanced Diet:** In remission, aim for a balanced diet rich in fruits, vegetables, lean proteins, and whole grains to maintain overall health.

◈ **Probiotics:** Some individuals find that probiotic supplements can help support gut health and reduce the risk of flares.

Special Diets (e.g., Low-Residue, Low-FODMAP):

1. Low-Residue Diet:

◈ This diet limits foods that are high in fibre and difficult to digest, making it easier on the digestive tract during flares.

◈ It includes white rice, refined pasta, well-cooked and peeled fruits and vegetables, and tender meats.

2. Low-FODMAP Diet:

◈ The low-FODMAP diet reduces foods high in fermentable carbohydrates (FODMAPs), which can trigger digestive symptoms.

◈ Common high-FODMAP foods include certain fruits, vegetables, legumes, and dairy products.

◈ This diet should be undertaken under the guidance of a healthcare provider or dietitian, as it requires careful planning to ensure nutritional adequacy.

Conclusion: Diet and nutrition are vital aspects of managing Crohn's Disease. Understanding dietary triggers, making adjustments during flares, and following special diets as needed can help individuals with Crohn's Disease reduce symptoms, promote healing, and maintain overall health. It is essential to work closely with healthcare providers and dietitians to develop a personalized nutrition plan tailored to the individual's specific needs and to ensure proper nutrient intake and symptom management.

Chapter 10: Lifestyle and Coping Strategies in Crohn's Disease

Living well with Crohn's Disease goes beyond medical treatments. This chapter explores the importance of managing stress, incorporating physical activity, and seeking support to enhance the overall quality of life for individuals with Crohn's Disease.

Managing Stress and Emotional Well-Being:

1. Understanding the Impact of Stress: Stress can exacerbate Crohn's Disease symptoms and trigger flares. It's essential to recognize the connection between emotional well-being and physical health.

2. Stress-Reduction Techniques: Strategies to manage stress include:

◇ **Mindfulness and Meditation:** These practices can help reduce anxiety and promote relaxation.

◇ **Deep Breathing Exercises:** Deep, slow breaths can calm the nervous system.

◇ **Yoga and Tai Chi:** These gentle forms of exercise incorporate relaxation techniques and can improve flexibility and balance.

◇ **Cognitive Behavioural Therapy (CBT):** CBT is a type of counselling that helps individuals identify and change negative thought patterns.

3. Seeking Support: Talking to a mental health professional or joining a support group can provide an outlet for discussing emotional challenges related to Crohn's Disease.

Exercise and Physical Activity:

1. Benefits of Exercise: Regular physical activity offers several advantages for individuals with Crohn's Disease:

◇ **Strengthening the Immune System:** Exercise can enhance immune function, potentially reducing the risk of infections.

◇ **Stress Reduction:** Physical activity releases endorphins, which can improve mood and reduce stress.

◇ **Maintaining Bone Health:** Weight-bearing exercises help maintain bone density, which can be affected by certain medications.

◇ **Enhancing Digestion:** Gentle exercises like walking can promote healthy digestion.

2. Tailoring Exercise: The type and intensity of exercise should be individualized based on one's overall health, fitness level, and current Crohn's Disease status. Consult with a healthcare provider or physical therapist for guidance.

3. Hydration: Staying well-hydrated is crucial during physical activity to prevent dehydration, which can be a concern for individuals with Crohn's Disease.

Support Networks and Counselling:

1. Peer Support Groups: Joining a Crohn's Disease support group can provide a sense of community, a platform for sharing experiences, and emotional support.

2. Family and Friends: Informing loved ones about the condition and its challenges can foster understanding and encourage a strong support system.

3. Professional Counselling: For individuals struggling with the emotional impact of Crohn's Disease, seeking counselling or therapy can be immensely helpful. Therapists can provide coping strategies and tools to manage stress, anxiety, and depression.

Conclusion:

Lifestyle and coping strategies are integral components of managing Crohn's Disease. By addressing stress, engaging in physical activity, and seeking support when needed, individuals with Crohn's Disease can improve their overall well-being and better navigate the challenges of living with a chronic condition. The holistic approach to managing Crohn's Disease includes not only medical treatments but also strategies to promote emotional and physical health, ultimately leading to a higher quality of life.

Chapter 11: Living with Crohn's Disease

Living with Crohn's Disease presents unique challenges, but with the right strategies and support, individuals can lead fulfilling lives. This chapter explores everyday challenges, coping mechanisms, balancing work, and social life, and traveling with Crohn's.

Everyday Challenges and Coping Mechanisms:

1. Fatigue: Managing chronic fatigue, a common symptom of Crohn's Disease, requires:

- Prioritizing rest and sleep.
- Establishing a regular sleep schedule.
- Listening to one's body and taking breaks when needed.

2. Abdominal Pain and Discomfort: Coping with pain includes:

- Taking medications as prescribed.
- Using heating pads or warm baths for relief.
- Practicing relaxation techniques to ease tension.

3. Dietary Restrictions: Adhering to dietary restrictions can be challenging. Coping mechanisms include:

- Planning meals in advance.
- Exploring alternative recipes.
- Consulting with a registered dietitian.

4. Frequent Bathroom Visits: Strategies for managing frequent trips to the restroom include:

- Familiarizing yourself with restroom locations in public places.
- Carrying a "restroom emergency" kit with supplies.

Balancing Work, Social Life, and Health:

1. Work-Life Balance: Achieving a work-life balance with Crohn's Disease involves:

◈ Open communication with employers about the condition.
◈ Requesting reasonable accommodations when necessary.
◈ Prioritizing self-care to prevent burnout.

2. Social Life: Maintaining an active social life while managing Crohn's Disease can be achieved through:

◈ Sharing your condition with friends and loved ones.
◈ Planning social events during periods of remission.
◈ Engaging in activities that accommodate your health needs.

3. Self-Care: Self-care is crucial for managing stress and maintaining health:

◈ Scheduling regular medical check-ups.
◈ Setting boundaries to protect your physical and emotional well-being.
◈ Engaging in hobbies and activities that bring joy and relaxation.

Traveling with Crohn's:

1. Pre-Trip Planning: When planning a trip, consider:

◈ Access to medical facilities at your destination.
◈ Medication needs and prescriptions.
◈ Dietary options and restrictions.
◈ The availability of restroom facilities.

2. Packing Essentials: Pack a travel kit that includes:

◇ Medications and necessary medical supplies.

◇ Snacks and bottled water.

◇ A change of clothes and personal hygiene items.

3. Communicate: Inform travel companions about your condition and needs, so they can provide support and understanding during the trip.

4. Plan Rest Stops: Plan for regular rest stops, especially during long journeys, to accommodate bathroom needs.

Conclusion:

Living with Crohn's Disease presents its share of challenges, but it is possible to lead a fulfilling life with the right strategies and support. By managing symptoms, balancing work, and social life, and planning ahead when traveling, individuals with Crohn's Disease can enjoy a high quality of life while effectively managing their condition. Remember that seeking support from healthcare providers, loved ones, and support groups can make a significant difference in navigating the journey of living with Crohn's Disease.

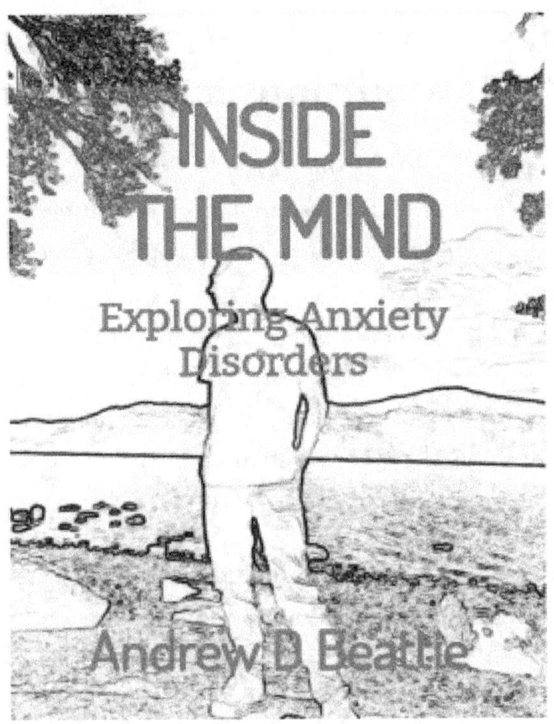
INSIDE
THE MIND
Exploring Anxiety
Disorders
Andrew D. Beattie

Chapter 12: Complications and Associated Conditions in Crohn's Disease

Crohn's Disease can lead to various complications and may be associated with other autoimmune and inflammatory conditions. This chapter explores fistulas and abscesses, strictures and obstructions, and these associated conditions.

Fistulas and Abscesses:

1. Fistulas: Fistulas are abnormal connections that can form between different parts of the digestive tract or between the digestive tract and other organs. They can be challenging to manage and may cause discomfort, infection, and complications.

⬦ **Symptoms:** Symptoms can include drainage of pus or stool from an opening near the anus, abdominal pain, and fever.

⬦ **Treatment:** Treatment often involves medications to control inflammation and infection, as well as surgical procedures to repair or divert the fistula.

2. Abscesses: Abscesses are pockets of pus that can develop within the abdominal cavity, often in association with fistulas or inflamed areas of the bowel.

⬦ **Symptoms:** Symptoms may include fever, severe abdominal pain, and a palpable mass in the abdomen.

⬦ **Treatment:** Abscesses typically require drainage, which may be performed through a needle aspiration or surgical procedure. Antibiotics are often prescribed to treat or prevent infection.

Strictures and Obstructions:

1. Strictures: Strictures are narrowed segments of the bowel caused by scarring and inflammation. They can lead to bowel obstructions, causing abdominal pain and vomiting.

◈ **Symptoms:** Symptoms of strictures may include cramping abdominal pain, bloating, and changes in bowel habits.

◈ **Treatment:** Treatment may involve medications to reduce inflammation and surgical intervention to remove or dilate strictures.

2. Bowel Obstructions: Complete blockages of the intestine can be painful and require immediate medical attention. Partial obstructions may resolve with conservative treatment.

◈ **Symptoms:** Symptoms include severe abdominal pain, vomiting, and a lack of bowel movements or gas.

◈ **Treatment:** Treatment varies depending on the severity of the obstruction and may include bowel rest, intravenous fluids, and surgical intervention if necessary.

Other Autoimmune and Inflammatory Conditions:
1. Arthritis: Some individuals with Crohn's Disease may develop arthritis, which can cause joint pain, stiffness, and swelling.

◈ **Treatment:** Treatment may involve medications to control inflammation and pain relief.

2. Skin Conditions: Conditions like erythema nodosum and pyoderma gangrenosum can manifest as painful skin lesions.

◈ **Treatment:** Treatment often includes medications to reduce inflammation and promote healing.

3. Eye Conditions: Uveitis and episcleritis are eye conditions that may occur in association with Crohn's Disease.

◇ **Treatment:** Treatment involves addressing the underlying inflammation and may include eye drops or other medications.

Conclusion:

Complications such as fistulas, abscesses, strictures, and bowel obstructions are possible in Crohn's Disease and require prompt medical attention. Additionally, individuals with Crohn's Disease should be aware of the potential for associated autoimmune and inflammatory conditions, which may require specialized care. Early detection, effective treatment, and ongoing monitoring are essential for managing these complications and associated conditions while maintaining a good quality of life.

Chapter 13: Paediatric and Adolescent Crohn's Disease

Diagnosing and managing Crohn's Disease in children and teenagers requires special attention to their unique needs and considerations. This chapter explores the challenges specific to paediatric and adolescent Crohn's Disease, as well as the transition to adult care.

Unique Considerations in Children and Teenagers:

1. Diagnosis Challenges: Diagnosing Crohn's Disease in children can be challenging because symptoms may overlap with other conditions, and children may have difficulty expressing their symptoms.

◇ Paediatric gastroenterologists are specialized in recognizing and diagnosing paediatric Crohn's Disease.

2. Growth and Development: Crohn's Disease can affect a child's growth and development due to malnutrition and inflammation. Monitoring growth and addressing nutritional needs are crucial.

3. Puberty: Adolescents with Crohn's Disease may face unique challenges during puberty, including delayed growth and sexual development. Managing symptoms and addressing nutritional deficiencies are vital.

4. Emotional and Social Impact: Adolescents may struggle with body image concerns, social isolation, and the emotional toll of living with a chronic condition. Psychosocial support and counselling can be beneficial.

5. School and Education: Frequent doctor's appointments and missed school days can impact a child's education. Communication between healthcare providers, schools, and parents is essential to ensure academic success.

Transitioning to Adult Care:

1. Timing of Transition: Transitioning from paediatric to adult care typically occurs between the ages of 18 and 21, depending on individual readiness and healthcare provider recommendations.

2. Preparing for Transition: The transition process involves:

⬧ Educating the adolescent about their condition, medications, and self-management.

⬧ Encouraging them to take a more active role in their healthcare.

⬧ Familiarizing them with adult healthcare providers and facilities.

3. Support During Transition: A transition coordinator or nurse can help facilitate the process and ensure continuity of care. Adolescents should be encouraged to ask questions and express their concerns.

4. Adult Care Considerations: Adult healthcare providers should be familiar with the unique challenges of Crohn's Disease in young adults and provide age-appropriate care.

Conclusion:

Diagnosing and managing Crohn's Disease in children and adolescents require a multidisciplinary approach that considers their unique physical, emotional, and social needs. The transition from paediatric to adult care is a significant milestone that should be carefully planned and executed to ensure seamless and comprehensive healthcare for young adults with Crohn's Disease. With proper support and guidance, children and teenagers living with Crohn's Disease can successfully manage their condition and lead fulfilling lives as they transition into adulthood.

Chapter 14: Research and Future Directions in Crohn's Disease (UK)

The United Kingdom has been at the forefront of Crohn's Disease research and innovation. This chapter explores ongoing research and clinical trials, promising treatments on the horizon, and the importance of patient advocacy and involvement in research.

Ongoing Research and Clinical Trials:

1. Academic Institutions: In the UK, renowned academic institutions, such as the University of Oxford, King's College London, and the University of Edinburgh, are conducting cutting-edge research on Crohn's Disease. Clinical trials are an essential part of this research landscape.

2. Biobanks: Biobanks like the UK IBD Genetics Consortium Biobank collect and store biological samples from individuals with Crohn's Disease. These resources support genetic and biomarker research.

3. National Health Service (NHS): The NHS plays a vital role in facilitating clinical trials and research studies related to Crohn's Disease. Patients often have the opportunity to participate in these trials, contributing to scientific advancements.

Promising Treatments on the Horizon:

1. Advanced Biologics: New biologic drugs with innovative mechanisms of action are being developed and tested. Some target specific molecules involved in inflammation, offering potential benefits over current treatments.

2. Personalized Medicine: Advances in genetics and biomarker research are leading to more personalized treatment approaches. Genetic profiling may help identify which medications are most effective for individual patients.

3. Microbiome Therapies: Research into the gut microbiome's role in Crohn's Disease has spurred interest in microbiome-based therapies, such as faecal microbiota transplantation (FMT) and microbiome-modulating drugs.

4. Stem Cell Therapies: Stem cell therapies are being explored as potential treatments for Crohn's Disease, with the goal of repairing damaged tissue and reducing inflammation.

Patient Advocacy and Involvement in Research:

1. Crohn's and Colitis UK: This patient advocacy organization in the UK actively supports and engages patients in research initiatives. They offer information, resources, and opportunities for patients to participate in clinical trials.

2. Patient-Cantered Research: The UK emphasizes patient-centred research, where the experiences and perspectives of individuals with Crohn's Disease are integrated into research design and decision-making.

3. Clinical Trial Participation: Patients are encouraged to consider participating in clinical trials, as this not only provides access to potentially groundbreaking treatments but also contributes to scientific progress.

4. Empowering Patients: Patient advocacy groups and healthcare providers empower individuals with Crohn's Disease to be active participants in their healthcare decisions and in shaping the future of research and treatment options.

Conclusion:

The United Kingdom is a hub of research and innovation in Crohn's Disease. Ongoing studies and clinical trials offer hope for improved treatments and better outcomes for individuals with Crohn's Disease. Patient advocacy and involvement in research play a crucial role in driving progress and ensuring that research efforts align with the needs and perspectives of those living with this condition. The future of Crohn's Disease management in the UK looks promising, with a focus on personalized medicine, innovative therapies, and active patient engagement in the research process.

Chapter 15: Resources and Support for Crohn's Disease

Individuals with Crohn's Disease can benefit from a wide range of resources and support networks. This chapter explores organizations and support groups, finding a healthcare team, and addressing financial and insurance considerations.

Organizations and Support Groups:

1. Crohn's and Colitis Foundation (UK): This nonprofit organization provides valuable resources, support, and information for individuals with Crohn's Disease and ulcerative colitis in the United Kingdom. They offer educational materials, advocacy efforts, and opportunities to connect with others through local chapters.

2. Crohn's and Colitis UK: This UK-based charity focuses on improving the lives of individuals affected by Crohn's Disease and ulcerative colitis. They offer support services, a helpline, and a wealth of information on managing these conditions.

3. Support Groups: Local support groups, often affiliated with national organizations, provide a safe space for individuals with Crohn's Disease to share experiences, seek advice, and build a sense of community.

Finding a Healthcare Team:

1. Gastroenterologist: A gastroenterologist is a medical specialist who diagnoses and treats gastrointestinal conditions, including Crohn's Disease. It's crucial to find a gastroenterologist with expertise in IBD.

2. Dietitian: A registered dietitian can provide guidance on managing dietary triggers and ensuring proper nutrition, which is vital for individuals with Crohn's Disease.

3. Psychologist or Therapist: Managing the emotional impact of Crohn's Disease is essential. A mental health professional can help individuals cope with stress, anxiety, and depression.

4. Primary Care Physician: A primary care doctor can coordinate overall healthcare, manage general health needs, and facilitate referrals to specialists.

Financial and Insurance Considerations:

1. Health Insurance: Understanding your health insurance coverage is crucial. Be aware of co-pays, deductibles, and coverage for medications and treatments. Consider seeking assistance from patient advocates or insurance specialists if needed.

2. Prescription Assistance Programs: Many pharmaceutical companies offer patient assistance programs that provide financial support or reduced costs for medications.

3. Employment and Disability: If Crohn's Disease affects your ability to work, explore options for short-term or long-term disability benefits, reasonable workplace accommodations, or assistance through government disability programs.

4. Financial Assistance: Some organizations, including patient advocacy groups, offer financial assistance programs to help with medical expenses, co-pays, and other related costs.

Conclusion:

Resources and support are essential components of effectively managing Crohn's Disease. National and local organizations, support groups, and a knowledgeable healthcare team can provide valuable guidance and assistance. Understanding your health insurance, exploring prescription assistance programs, and addressing financial considerations are also critical to ensure that healthcare needs are met without undue financial burden. By accessing these resources and building a strong support network, individuals with Crohn's Disease can better navigate the challenges of living with a chronic condition and improve their overall quality of life.

Chapter 16: Personal Stories and Inspirational Accounts

Real-life stories of individuals living with Crohn's Disease provide valuable insights into the triumphs and challenges they face. These accounts offer encouragement and inspiration to those navigating their own journeys with this chronic condition.

1. Triumphs and Challenges:

Living with Crohn's Disease presents a unique set of challenges, but it also showcases incredible resilience and determination. Here are some personal stories of individuals who have faced the ups and downs of Crohn's Disease:

- **Sarah's Story:** Sarah was diagnosed with Crohn's Disease at a young age, and she struggled with frequent flares and hospitalizations. Despite the challenges, she found strength in her supportive family and friends. Through trial and error, she discovered dietary strategies that worked for her and allowed her to regain control of her life. Sarah's story is a testament to perseverance and the importance of a strong support network.

- **James's Journey:** James was an avid athlete before his Crohn's Disease diagnosis. The initial shock of the diagnosis forced him to adjust his lifestyle, but it didn't dampen his competitive spirit. He gradually returned to sports and even completed a marathon to raise awareness for Crohn's Disease research. James's journey reminds us that with determination, it's possible to pursue your passions despite the obstacles.

- **Emma's Empowerment:** Emma's journey with Crohn's Disease led her to become an advocate for others. She joined patient support groups, participated in clinical trials, and shared her experiences through a blog. Her advocacy work not only raised awareness about Crohn's Disease but also empowered others to take control of their health and seek the best possible care.

2. Words of Encouragement:

Living with Crohn's Disease can be challenging, but these inspirational accounts offer words of encouragement to those on a similar path:

⬦ "In the face of adversity, we discover our inner strength. Crohn's Disease may test us, but it doesn't define us. Keep pushing forward, and you'll find that you're capable of more than you ever imagined."

⬦ "Remember, you're not alone in this journey. There is a supportive community of fellow Crohn's warriors who understand what you're going through. Lean on them for guidance, empathy, and friendship."

⬦ "Every day with Crohn's Disease is a victory. Celebrate the small wins, whether it's a symptom-free day or successfully managing a flare-up. Each step forward is a testament to your resilience."

Glossary of Medical Terms and Jargon:

This glossary aims to clarify medical terms and jargon frequently encountered when dealing with Crohn's Disease:

1. **Inflammation:** The body's response to injury or infection, often characterized by redness, swelling, pain, and heat.

2. **Colonoscopy:** A medical procedure that involves examining the colon and rectum using a flexible tube with a camera.

3. **Endoscopy:** A procedure using a thin, flexible tube with a camera to visualize the inside of the digestive tract.

4. **Biopsy:** The removal of a small sample of tissue for examination under a microscope to diagnose or monitor diseases.

5. **Remission:** A period during which the symptoms of Crohn's Disease are controlled or absent.

6. **Flare-Up:** A sudden and severe worsening of Crohn's Disease symptoms.

7. **Immunosuppressants:** Medications that suppress the immune system to reduce inflammation.

8. **Fistula:** An abnormal connection that can form between organs or between the digestive tract and the skin.

9. **Obstruction:** A blockage that prevents the normal flow of food and fluids through the intestine.

10. **Microbiome:** The community of microorganisms, including bacteria, living in the gut.

Appendix: Additional Resources, Websites, and Books:

The following resources, websites, and books provide valuable information and support for individuals with Crohn's Disease and their caregivers:

Websites and Online Resources:

◈ **Crohn's and Colitis Foundation (UK):** Website[1]

◈ Offers comprehensive information, support, and resources for individuals with Crohn's Disease and ulcerative colitis in the UK.

◈ **NHS Crohn's Disease Information:** Website[2]

◈ Provides NHS-approved information on Crohn's Disease, including symptoms, treatments, and self-help tips.

◈ **Crohn's Forum:** Website[3]

◈ An online community where individuals with Crohn's Disease can connect, share experiences, and seek advice.

Recommended Books:

◈ "Living with Crohn's & Colitis: A Comprehensive Naturopathic Guide for Complete Digestive Wellness" by Dede Cummings and Jessica Black.

---

1. https://www.crohnsandcolitis.org.uk/

2. https://www.nhs.uk/conditions/crohns-disease/

3. https://www.crohnsforum.com/

◇ A guidebook that explores natural approaches to managing Crohn's Disease and colitis.

◇ "Breaking the Vicious Cycle: Intestinal Health Through Diet" by Elaine Gottschall.

◇ Offers insights into the Specific Carbohydrate Diet (SCD), which some individuals with Crohn's Disease find helpful.

◇ "The First Year: Crohn's Disease and Ulcerative Colitis: An Essential Guide for the Newly Diagnosed" by Jill Sklar and Ann Steinhart.

◇ A practical guide for those recently diagnosed with Crohn's Disease or ulcerative colitis.

Conclusion:

This Glossary and Appendix section aims to enhance your understanding of Crohn's Disease-related terminology and provide a curated list of resources, websites, and recommended books. Whether you are seeking clarity on medical terms or looking for additional information and support, these resources are designed to assist you on your Crohn's Disease journey.

Chapter 17: Misdiagnosis in Crohn's Disease

Receiving a correct diagnosis is a crucial first step in effectively managing Crohn's Disease. However, the journey to diagnosis can sometimes be fraught with challenges, including the risk of misdiagnosis. This chapter explores the causes, consequences, and prevention of misdiagnosis in Crohn's Disease.

Causes of Misdiagnosis:

Misdiagnosis can occur in various medical conditions, including Crohn's Disease, and can result from several factors:

1. **Symptom Overlap:** Crohn's Disease shares symptoms with other gastrointestinal disorders, such as irritable bowel syndrome (IBS) or celiac disease. The similarity in symptoms can lead to confusion.

2. **Atypical Presentations:** Some individuals with Crohn's Disease may exhibit atypical symptoms or patterns of inflammation that don't fit the typical diagnostic criteria.

3. **Inconsistent Symptoms:** Crohn's Disease can have periods of remission, during which symptoms subside. If a patient is in remission during a doctor's visit, it may lead to a misdiagnosis or delayed diagnosis.

4. **Lack of Awareness:** Healthcare providers who are less familiar with Crohn's Disease may not consider it as a potential diagnosis, especially when symptoms are subtle or not well-documented.

Consequences of Misdiagnosis:

Misdiagnosis in Crohn's Disease can have several significant consequences:

1. **Delayed Treatment:** A misdiagnosis can result in a delay in receiving appropriate treatment. This delay may allow the disease to progress, leading to more severe symptoms and complications.

2. **Unnecessary Treatments:** In some cases, individuals may receive treatments for conditions they don't have, which can lead to unnecessary medical procedures and medications.

3. **Psychological Impact:** The uncertainty and frustration of being misdiagnosed can take a toll on a patient's mental well-being, causing anxiety and emotional distress.

4. **Financial Burden:** Misdiagnosis can result in costly medical bills, including unnecessary tests, procedures, and medications.

Prevention and Seeking a Second Opinion:
To reduce the risk of misdiagnosis and ensure a correct diagnosis of Crohn's Disease, consider the following steps:

1. **Consult a Specialist:** Seek care from a gastroenterologist, who specializes in digestive disorders and is more likely to recognize the signs of Crohn's Disease.

2. **Provide a Detailed Medical History:** Be thorough in describing your symptoms, their duration, and any family history of gastrointestinal disorders.

3. **Ask for Additional Testing:** If initial tests are inconclusive, don't hesitate to request further diagnostic procedures, such as endoscopy, colonoscopy, or imaging studies.

4. Seek a Second Opinion: If you suspect a misdiagnosis or feel uncertain about your diagnosis, consider seeking a second opinion from another healthcare provider or specialist.

5. Advocate for Yourself: Be an active advocate for your health. If you believe you have Crohn's Disease but haven't received a diagnosis, express your concerns to your healthcare provider and ask for further evaluation.

Chapter 18: Mental Health Challenges in Crohn's Disease

Living with Crohn's Disease brings not only physical challenges but also profound emotional and psychological impacts. In this chapter, we explore the mental health challenges that individuals with Crohn's Disease may face and strategies for coping with them.

Understanding the Emotional Impact:

The emotional toll of Crohn's Disease can be significant and multifaceted. It's essential to recognize and acknowledge the following emotional challenges:

1. **Anxiety:** The unpredictability of flare-ups, symptoms, and treatment outcomes can lead to heightened anxiety levels.

2. **Depression:** The chronic nature of the condition, along with pain and fatigue, can contribute to feelings of hopelessness and depression.

3. **Stress:** Coping with the daily demands of managing a chronic illness can lead to chronic stress, affecting overall well-being.

4. **Isolation:** Fear of symptoms or embarrassment may lead individuals to isolate themselves, impacting their social lives and mental health.

Impact on Quality of Life:

Mental health challenges can significantly affect the quality of life for individuals with Crohn's Disease:

◈ **Reduced Quality of Life:** Untreated mental health issues can lead to decreased overall quality of life, affecting relationships, work, and daily activities.

◈ **Worsening Symptoms:** High-stress levels and mental health struggles can exacerbate Crohn's Disease symptoms, creating a vicious cycle.

Coping Strategies:

To address the mental health challenges associated with Crohn's Disease, consider implementing the following coping strategies:

1. **Seek Professional Help:** Consult a mental health professional, such as a therapist or counsellor, who can provide support and therapeutic interventions tailored to your needs.

2. **Build a Support Network:** Share your feelings and experiences with friends and family who can provide emotional support and understanding.

3. **Mindfulness and Relaxation:** Practice mindfulness techniques, meditation, or deep breathing exercises to reduce stress and anxiety.

4. **Balanced Lifestyle:** Prioritize self-care, including adequate sleep, a balanced diet, and regular exercise to support both physical and mental well-being.

5. **Support Groups:** Join a Crohn's Disease support group or online community to connect with others who share similar experiences.

6. **Open Communication:** Discuss your mental health concerns with your healthcare team, as they can provide guidance and resources for managing both your physical and emotional health.

Reducing Stigma:

Reducing the stigma associated with mental health challenges is essential. By openly discussing mental health, we can create a more supportive and understanding environment for individuals with Crohn's Disease.

Conclusion:

Managing Crohn's Disease is not only about addressing physical symptoms but also addressing the mental health challenges that can arise. By acknowledging these challenges, seeking support, and implementing effective coping strategies, individuals with Crohn's Disease can improve their overall quality of life and well-being. Remember that you are not alone in facing these challenges, and there is help and support available to navigate the emotional aspects of living with Crohn's Disease.

Conclusion:

Navigating the Crohn's Journey

In your journey through the pages of "All About Crohn's Disease," you've explored the intricacies of this chronic condition, from its definition to its diagnosis, treatment, and beyond. Crohn's Disease, with its unique challenges and complexities, may have seemed daunting at times, but it's essential to remember that knowledge is power.

Empowerment Through Knowledge:

Understanding Crohn's Disease is the first step in taking control of your health. You've delved into the details of its symptoms, diagnostic processes, and treatment options, gaining insights into the management of flare-ups, dietary considerations, and the importance of a supportive network. Armed with this knowledge, you are better equipped to navigate the uncertainties of life with Crohn's Disease.

The Strength Within:

Throughout this book, you've encountered the inspiring stories of individuals who've faced the triumphs and challenges that Crohn's Disease can present. Their stories serve as a reminder that resilience, determination, and the support of friends, family, and healthcare providers can help you overcome the hurdles along your own journey.

Looking Ahead:

As research continues and medical advancements evolve, the landscape of Crohn's Disease management is ever-changing. Stay informed, engage with your healthcare team, and consider participating in research efforts to contribute to the ongoing progress in the field.

You're Not Alone:

Remember that you're not alone on this path. There are organizations, support groups, and fellow individuals with Crohn's Disease who understand and empathize with your experiences. Seek out these communities, both online and in your local area, for shared wisdom, guidance, and camaraderie.

A Brighter Tomorrow:

Though Crohn's Disease may present its challenges, it does not define you. With knowledge, support, and determination, you can lead a fulfilling life, pursuing your passions, and achieving your goals. The future holds promise for better treatments, increased understanding, and improved quality of life for those living with Crohn's Disease.

Thank you for embarking on this educational journey with "All About Crohn's Disease." May it serve as a valuable resource, a source of empowerment, and a beacon of hope as you continue your path toward a brighter, healthier tomorrow.

Wishing you strength, resilience, and good health on your journey with Crohn's Disease.

Visit my Online Store

All of my books are available to download in pdf format on my website:

www.AndrewDBeattie.co.uk

or search for "Andrew D Beattie" at the following :

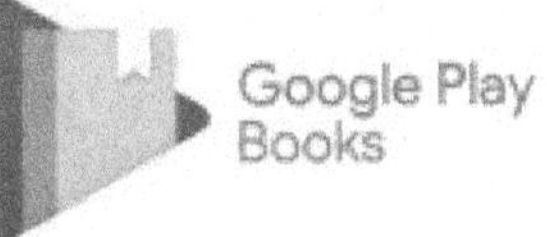
Books
Google Play
Books

Don't miss out!

Visit the website below and you can sign up to receive emails whenever Andrew D Beattie publishes a new book. There's no charge and no obligation.

https://books2read.com/r/B-A-MYHZ-CNSOC

BOOKS 2 READ

Connecting independent readers to independent writers.

Did you love *All About Crohn's Disease*? Then you should read *A - Z of Mental Health*[1] by Andrew D Beattie!

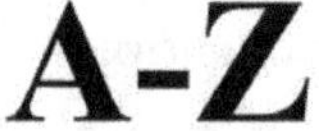

Of Mental Health

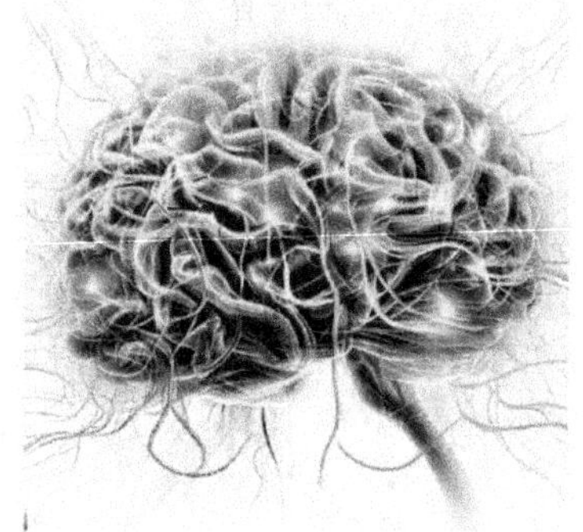

Andrew D Beattie

2

Navigating the maze of mental health can be a complex and overwhelming experience. "A - Z of Mental Health" serves as a comprehensive guide that breaks down the labyrinth into manageable pieces. Whether you're a patient seeking to understand your own mind, a loved one looking to support someone you care about, or a healthcare provider wanting to improve your practice, this book provides valuable insights for all.

Inside these pages, you will find:

Alphabetically-Organized Entries: From Anxiety Disorders to Zoloft, easily find and understand a vast array of terms related to mental health.

---

1. https://books2read.com/u/3GGzgO

2. https://books2read.com/u/3GGzgO

In-Depth Explanations: Each term is accompanied by a thorough explanation that breaks down the complexities of conditions and treatments.

Resource Directories: Comprehensive lists of helplines, organizations, and support groups within the UK, including specific resources for Scotland.

Legal and Ethical Context: Important information about the UK laws that affect mental health care, including confidentiality, involuntary commitment, and the rights of the mentally ill.

Designed to be accessible, "A - Z of Mental Health" dispels myths, educates, and empowers. In a society where mental health remains stigmatized and misunderstood, this book aims to bring clarity and support to those who need it most.